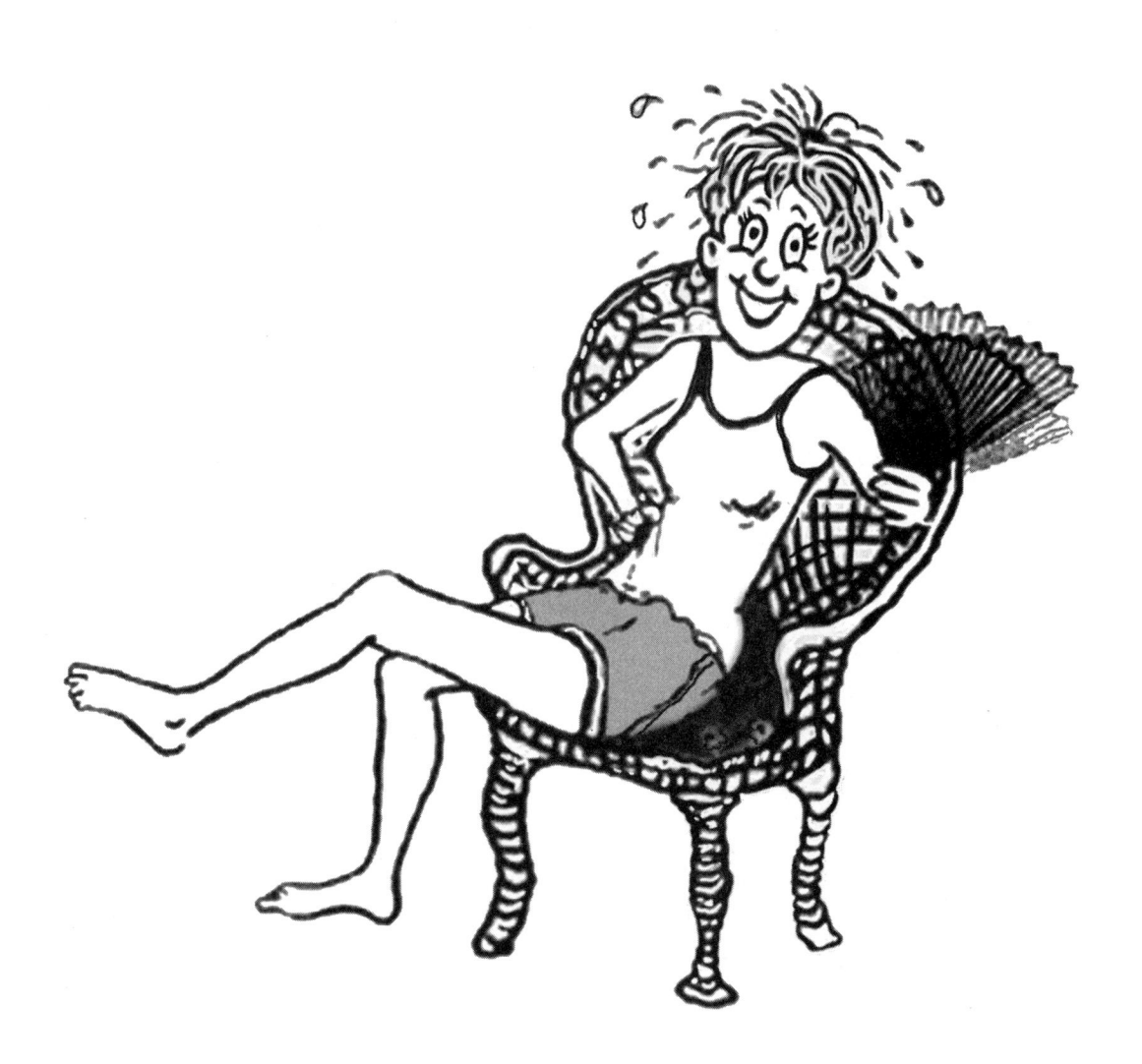

IS IT HOT IN HERE...
OR IS IT ME?

Mastering the Maze of Menopause

Indus Publishing Corporation
Wayland, New York

IS IT HOT IN HERE...
OR IS IT ME?

Mastering the Maze of Menopause

by

Lorraine D'Abate

and

Nancy Kenyon

Illustrations by John Blakely

Published by Indus Publishing Corporation

Indus Publishing Corporation
7052 Pokey Moonshine
Wayland, New York 14572
Fax: 716-728-9756

Copyright © 2000 by Lorraine D'Abate & Nancy Kenyon
    Indus Publishing Corporation
    All Publishing, distribution, and licensing for
    all media - Indus Publishing Corporation

All rights reserved under International and Pan-American Copyright

Reproduction or translation of any part of this work beyond permitted by Section 107 or 108 of the 1976 United Sates Copyright Act without the permission of the copyright owner is unlawful. Requests for permission or further information should be addressed to the Permission Department, Indus Publishing.

Limits of Liability and Disclaimer of Warranty
The author is solely responsible for the contents of this book, expressed or implied. The publishers are indemnified against liability in any form of content or presentation.

ISBN: 1-890838-03-9
Library of Congress: 00-105016

Other Books By Indus Publishing

The Non-Trivial Trivia Book
Control Yourself!
The Complete Guide To Foreign Medical Schools
MCAT: The Answer Key
SAT I: The Answer Key
One Track

VIII

DEDICATION

For HELEN JUDD
A great inspiration and role model.

TABLE OF CONTENTS

CHAPTER	PAGE
Introduction	1
1. Color Me Red	5
2. Fuzzy Wuzzy Wasn't Just a Bear	9
3. Night Sweats	13
4. Best Foot Forward (Not!)	17
5. Tossin' and Turnin'	21
6. Memory Loss	25
7. Blue is Just Another Color	27
8. You Are What You Think	31
9. Slowly I Turn	35
10. Who Me?	39
11. Read it and Bleep @#$&*	43

CHAPTER	PAGE
12. Get Real!	47
13. Mirror, Mirror on the Wall	51
14. More on Memory Loss	55
15. Larger Than Life	59
16. Hair Today, Hair Tomorrow	63
17. To Each Her Own	67
18. A River Runs Through It	69
19. Do You See What I See?	73
20. Mall Madness	77
21. School Daze	81
22. Soft Shoe for the Soul	85
23. Wrap Up	89

INTRODUCTION

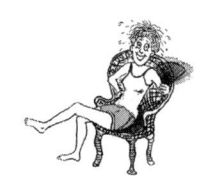

Your 50-year old cousin looks like hell, but you don't look a day over 40. Sound familiar?

In the next decade, over 43 million women will reach menopause. And, it appears from most popular literature on the subject, that many of us are in a pathological state of denial.

We cling to the image of ourselves as 30-year olds. We spend enough money on face creams to sponsor a Little League team; enough hours reading articles about "beating the clock" (whether through exercise, diet or cosmetic surgery) to have mastered a foreign language. Hey, wait a minute! Let's get a grip. We ARE middle-aged; we will never be 30 years old again. Let's face it, in some ways it's a blessing.

We deprive ourselves, and our sisters who come after us, of fully experiencing the most profound change since puberty. Let's not treat menopause like some book that should be carried around in a brown wrapper. Let's get it out of the wrapper, put it on the table and get familiar with its contents.

The important thing is to recognize the symptoms of menopause and educate ourselves on ways to treat these symptoms, whether through physician care, reading material on the subject, hormone replacement, herbal therapies, acupuncture, diet, massage, blah, blah, blah. What matters is choosing a course of action which works for us as individuals. But guess what? These actions may provide an easier passage, but pass we must. All the estrogen, tofu and oysters in the world will not return us to our 20's.

The most important factors in coping with menopause are loving, caring for and understanding ourselves... and having A SENSE OF HUMOR. You see, ultimately, most of what we consider great human drama is, on the flip side, great human comedy. Seeing our reflection in a store window and stopping to wonder how our heads got on our mothers' bodies can be a very tragic or hysterically comic moment (not to mention the mileage you can get out of the story).

Let's stop saying to each other, as the highest form of compliment, "You look so young"—and start being honest. We have an opportunity now to make a real growth spurt, leave behind the physical dreams of youth, and embrace an image of ourselves as wise, experienced and full of mirth.

Let's lighten up. We'll give you some hints for coping with menopause that are working for us. The whole process has real entertainment value which is our purpose in writing this book. We hope you will enjoy reading it as much as we have enjoyed writing it. We are women in transition and we call ourselves WITS.

"When I want GOOD work done, I look about me for a woman over 45."
M. Harland

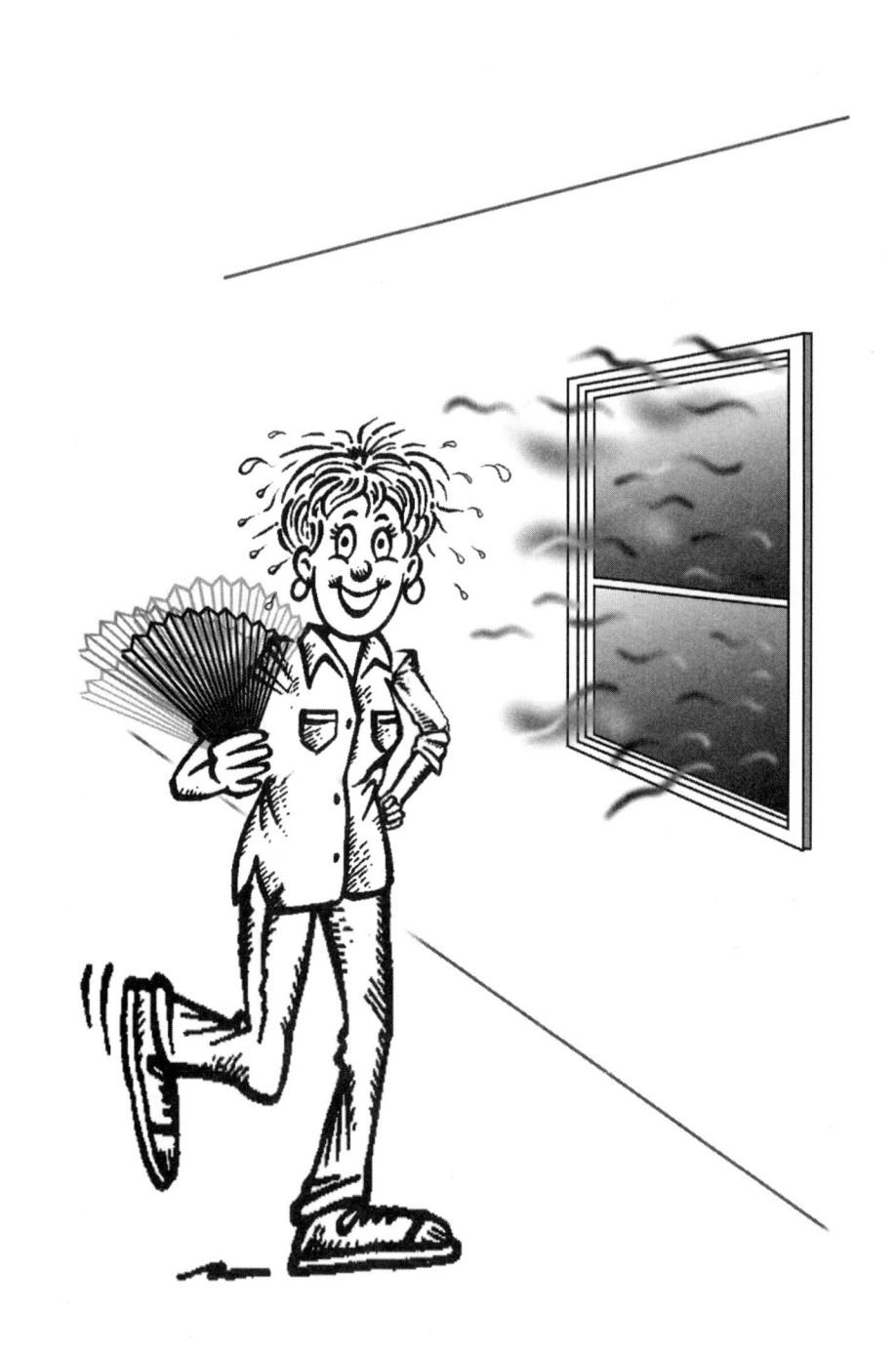

1

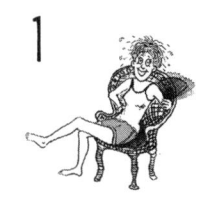

COLOR ME RED

When ANYONE mentions menopause, "hot flash" is the most talked about symptom. We prefer to call them "power surges". These surges are experienced by about 80% of menopausal women. You know, those Women in Transition/WITS. Generally, but not necessarily, these surges begin in the chest, spread to the neck, always the face and sometimes the arms. They are often accompanied by beads of sweat that rival the Chinese water torture. Those of you who have been there already know what we're talking about. You know, when your body temperature goes from 98.6 to 127 degrees in 7 seconds: A real trip to Bizarro World.

Not long ago, some of our friends started a monthly card game. It's a friendly game that consists of a lot of eating, talking and laughing. And, oh yes, some card playing. It doesn't make a difference if it's winter or summer, when before long someone exclaims, "Is it hot"... (you know the rest). While windows are thrown open, Helen, age 80, sits looking quite contentedly—in her sweater—with an all-knowing smile on her face. She's paid her dues. She's been there, done that.

As for the rest of the card players, who are only beginning the passage, conversation naturally turns to power surge stories. Mary says that by the time she makes up in the morning, she has already experienced no less than three hot flashes. Her old solution was a mad dash to the car, turn on the air conditioning and attempt to restore a make-up job that was reminiscent of wax dripping down a candle. Her approach has now changed. Because it's an exercise in futility to make up at home, she does full face make up in the car these days. Hey, it works!

We all have many stories about where, when and how we've surged. Too bad we're not always among friends when our surges decide to take over. It's hard to be nonchalant when your face is bright red and you're sweating bullets.

Recently, Joyce surged at a wedding reception. Fortunately, most of the wedding guests were doing some very vigorous folk dances (Hora, Tarantella, etc.). When asked if she was okay, it was quite easy to reply that she had just put in a rigorous 20-minute set of dancing herself. After taking a short break, she would be back on the floor.

The same situation (dreaded red face/sweating bullets routine) is not quite so easy when making a business presentation. Not to worry, there are options there as well:

> If close to 50% of the group are women, a simple "Is it hot in here…" will suffice. The women will all laugh. Even if it's not their particular problem at present, the older ones will remember, and the younger ones will want to be part of the club. The men will laugh just to be hip.

> If this is not comfortable or quite your style, then act so excited about what you're presenting that the audience will be convinced it's manifesting itself physically. Use any of the following phrases: "Now we're cooking." "This product is hot." "A virtual fire sale." "Will sell like hot cakes."

Or how about, keep tugging at your collar and whisper (loud enough for everyone to hear), "Collar too tight." Then, intermittently, stretch your neck as if trying to wriggle away from the collar.

If all else fails, keep repeating to yourself, "Don't sweat the small stuff." Get it??

As we go through this passage of our lives, our mutual mantra being "Is It hot...", remember we have options:

Keep home and workplace cool.

Dress in loose, layered clothing which can be easily removed.

Drink plenty of water.

Fight with everyone about thermostat control.

Take karate lessons so that you alone can commandeer the thermostat at work.

At home, control of the thermostat is simpler—just scream a lot. It's so attractive and feminine.

Join a nudist colony (preferably in Alaska).

"The greater part of our happiness or misery depends on our dispositions and not on our circumstances."
Martha Washington

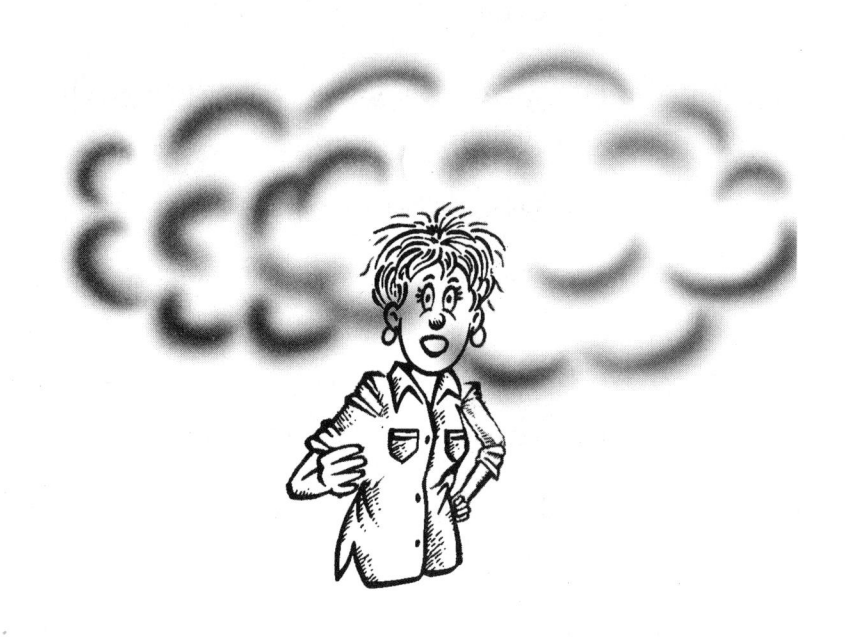

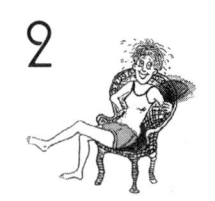

FUZZY WUZZY WAS NOT JUST A BEAR

Fuzzy thinking can be expressed in one word: Cottonhead.

This is the feeling of being adrift in your own brain, disorganized, unable to assemble thoughts and loss of verbal expression.

If you are experiencing any or all of the above, not to worry. These are common physical symptoms of menopause. Cottonhead means the left brain stuff, which controls logic and intellectual thinking, is temporarily impaired.

Take the case of the weekly planner. This organizational tool is virtually useless if you can't remember what day it is or where you put it. Paying bills on time can't happen if you're constantly depositing them in the trash along with your junk mail. And how can you straighten out your landlord if you can't remember his name or where he lives? Cottonhead rules—but opportunity has knocked. Don't fight it! Revel in it. See it as a vacation from words, definition and direction. In fact, we're in Cottonhead now.

We are forced into our right brains which control the heart and creative thinking. This actually can be a lovely part of the brain to visit. Here we can withdraw from the world ruled by the steely, organized intellect and experience ourselves differently. It's a good time to explore other facets of our lives.

This is the time to let your spirit flow freely, daydream (napping doesn't count), meditate and see where your intuition takes you. There's no special place to do this. It's your choice—the beach, a lake, the mountains, the desert, your own imagination.

Your right brain is always with you. In this altered state, many women have made positive changes. Celebrate this wake up call.

"It's all part of life's rich pageant; I wouldn't change a thing."
T. Martin

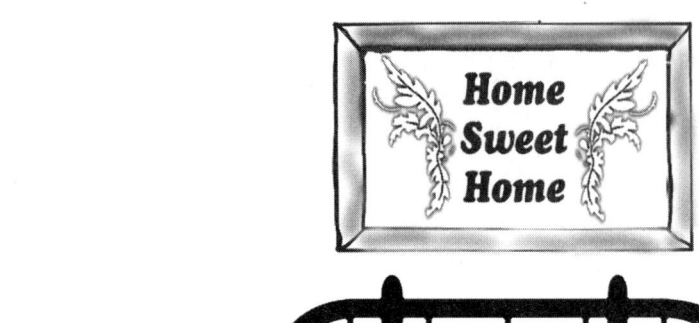

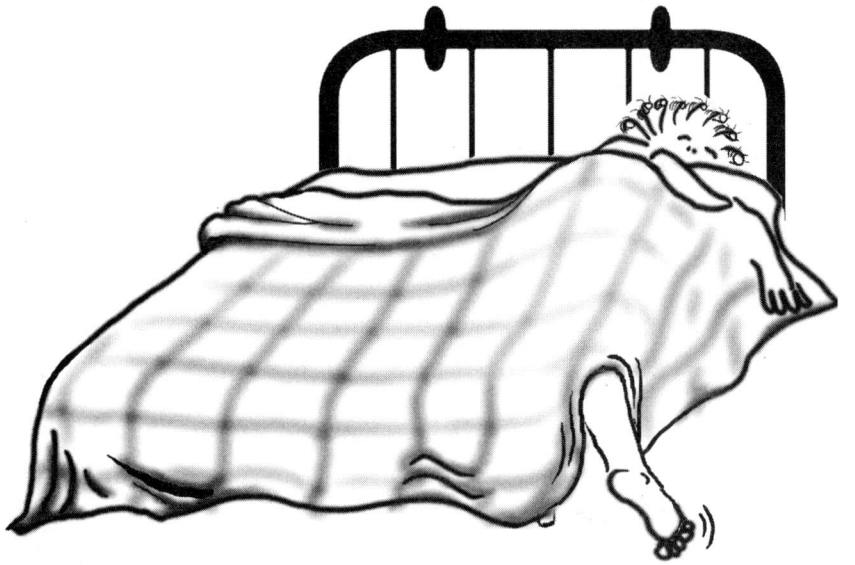

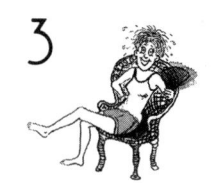

NIGHT SWEATS

Cathy tells of the winter night she went to bed. You know the look —red plaid flannel nightgown, little white tennis booties edged in pink, and yellow velcro rollers on the top and sides of her head. She awoke the following morning totally nude. Go figure.

Her best guess is that it was NIGHT SWEATS. The nightgown was on the floor at the foot of the bed, the socks were thrown on both sides of the bed. The velcro rollers were tossed around the bedroom. She's confident that only one is still missing. It will probably show up when she cleans the ceiling light fixture or runs the ceiling fan.

Night sweats represent more than throwing off blankets, soaking the sheets, changing the linens and nightgown. Let's say it represents the process by which Ma Nature cleanses us. The inner furnace is suddenly stoked. The purpose in building up the fires is to purify us while releasing toxins, both physical and psychological. This purification is reminiscent of the Native American sweat lodge. It allows us to tap new psychic resources.

Who needs years of psychoanalysis when we can sweat out our fears? Instead of complaining to other WITS about these night sweats, how about bragging "Hey, last night I sweated out not being chosen as a cheerleader in high school" or "I no longer care that the sun streaks in my hair are gray" or "Who cares that I wore white shoes after Labor Day."

In the meantime, while you're waiting for all your wisdom to arrive, keep lots of water on your night stand and a change of clothes next to the bed. Be sure to use one foot as the thermostat for your body. For some magical reason, simply dangling one foot from the side of the bed cools the body. We don't know why, but it works.

"Life can only be understood backward, but must be lived forward."
Soren Kierkegaard

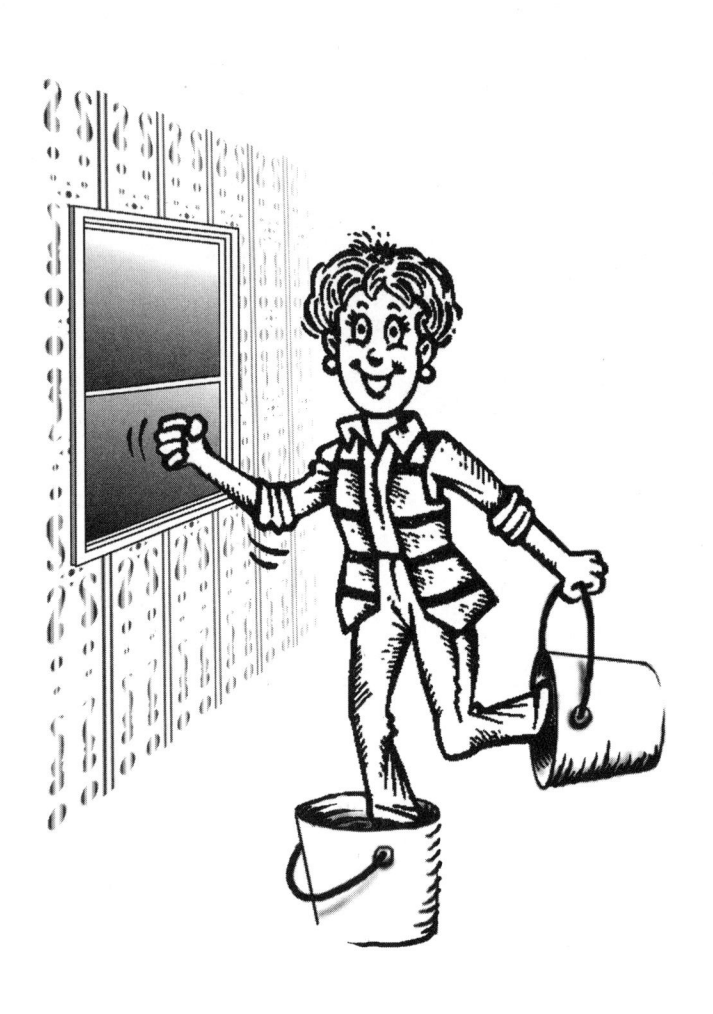

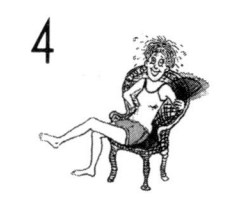

BEST FOOT FORWARD (NOT!)

Sweaty feet. Yet another not-so-attractive symptom lurking in menopause's bag of tricks.

Debbie, who recently turned 45, has been experiencing menopausal symptoms for about a year and handles them with good grace.

One day while teaching Spanish class, Debbie remarked to her students that there was a particularly foul odor in the room. One student, who had a crush on her, was determined to find the cause. The best he could do was pinpoint it to something under her desk. She suspected a dead rodent under the floor boards and intended to report it to maintenance. However, on the way home, she noticed the same odor in her car. Later, she detected this same foul odor in her bed. Aha! The culprits were her own odoriferous feet.

Smelly feet are accompanied by the constant feeling of walking around in water buckets. That "squish, squish" sound is NOT a pursuing swamp monster.

Solutions:

    Wear sandals.

    Go barefoot.

    Keep all shoes in the freezer.

We don't need no stinkin' feet.

"You never know another person until you walk in their shoes."
Mom

Sleepy Times Holodeck

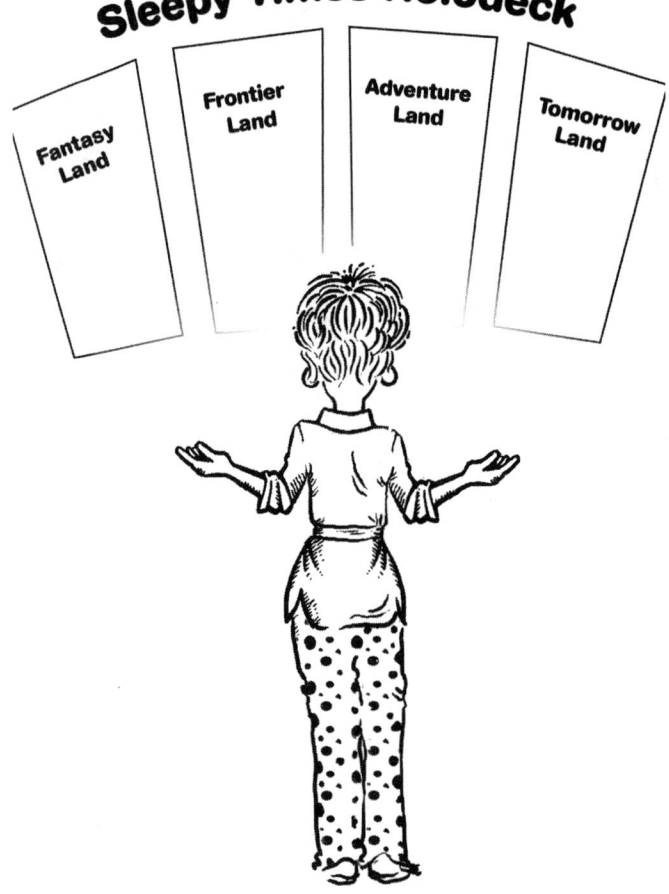

- Fantasy Land
- Frontier Land
- Adventure Land
- Tomorrow Land

5

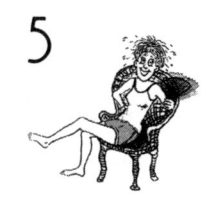

TOSSIN' & TURNIN'

Just when we begin to love the notion of sleep, our bodies decide 47 minutes of rest at a time is enough. You know the drill. Exhausted after a long day, you climb into bed, cover yourself with five quilts and begin to doze. Suddenly, your body temperature shoots up 15 degrees and the quilts go flying. Off with the socks and the jammies. You are wide awake. The fat around your hips begins to take on a life of its own. You feel it spreading and pressing into the mattress. Then the brain begins spinning scenarios of past and future disasters. Your hands are clasped in tight little balls, teeth gnashing. Welcome to menopause.

It is difficult to find the upside to these bouts of sleeplessness. Yet, there must be a way we can make this physical phenomena work for us. (Getting up to eat is not an option nor is reliving the death of your beloved dog.)

Pick up any woman's magazine and it is full of suggestions for dealing with sleeplessness: relaxation techniques; reading in another room; no sugar or caffeine. All of these solutions have merit, but are they fun? We have come up with an approach which may make these sleepless hours actually entertaining.

We propose traveling. Not in a car or plane, but psychic traveling. Just imagine the Women in Transition equivalent to the Star Trek Holodeck, except all the action takes place in your imagination.

Remember The Wonderful World of Disney which aired Sunday nights on TV back in the 1950's? Reconstructing a mental world based on this program is guaranteed to turn sleeplessness into an adventure in creative visualization, with no commercials.

With eyes closed and body relaxed, enter your own Disneyland. In front of you is a choice of four doors: Adventure Land, Frontier Land, Tomorrow Land and Fantasy Land. Open the door of your choice and step into a world created completely by your imagination.

Okay, so you choose Adventure Land. Picture every detail. What are you wearing? No doubt, a safari hat, super cool leather boots, 100% cotton culottes and, of course, a safari jacket. Perhaps you are going to live among the gorillas or start a school in Uganda. Feel the hot sun on your face, experience the sense of excitement and commitment as you set off in your jeep across the Savannah. Adventure awaits! If you happen to doze off before you reach your destination, you can always pick up where you left off next time insomnia strikes.

Maybe you prefer Frontier Land where women of strength and endurance made their mark. Turn the knob, enter the great American wilderness, and begin to bend circumstances of great challenge to your will. Are you a member of a group of settlers making the great trek westward in search of a new beginning? Perhaps you are a member of the Donner party and, hopefully, a healthy vegetarian. You carry little Johnny across the pass just because you can. Feel his weight on your shoulders as you plod through waist-high snow. Experience the majestic loneliness of the Rockies as you continue on and on and on. (You're getting tired now. Your eyes are growing heavy—you are sinking into sleep. Night, night.)

The next time you are lying bug-eyed in bed, you may wish to visit Tomorrow Land. You turn the knob and step into your ideal future. Feel your good health and enthusiasm. You have become your actualized self, full of confidence and good will. Whether you are growing prize-winning tomatoes or dressing for a book signing at Barnes & Noble, you are glad to be you. Hey, this is fun!

Fantasy Land is your own business. Just make it last.

Please note: There is no Yesterday Land. Spending sleepless hours mucking around in the past is guaranteed to leave you emotionally hung over in the morning. What's done is done. Our pasts all contain regrets and losses. Only the very adept psychic traveler can visit the past and come back refreshed.

There are a few rules. Never, never conjure up an unhappy ending. Never, never hurt yourself or others. This is about creating lovely pictures and good karma.

The next time you are lying in bed listening to the clock tick, take a very deep breath and step onto your own private Holodeck. Here all good things are possible. You create, produce and direct a reverie starring your best self. It's your movie, make it a blockbuster. Eventually, the line between your images and your dreams will dissolve. You'll be snoring before you know it, AND you'll wake up happy in the morning.

"Imagination is the highest kite one can fly."
We forget who said this.

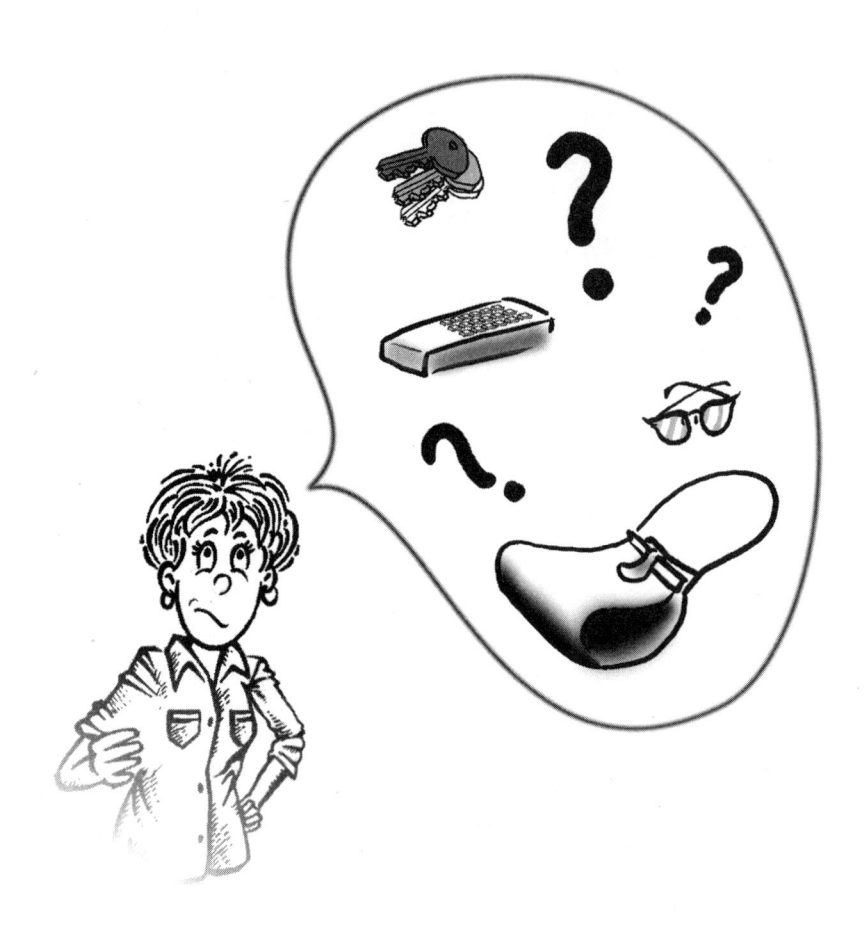

6

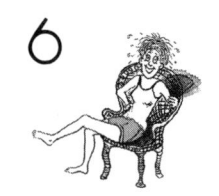

MEMORY LOSS

"We'll have these moments to remember."
The Four Somebodies

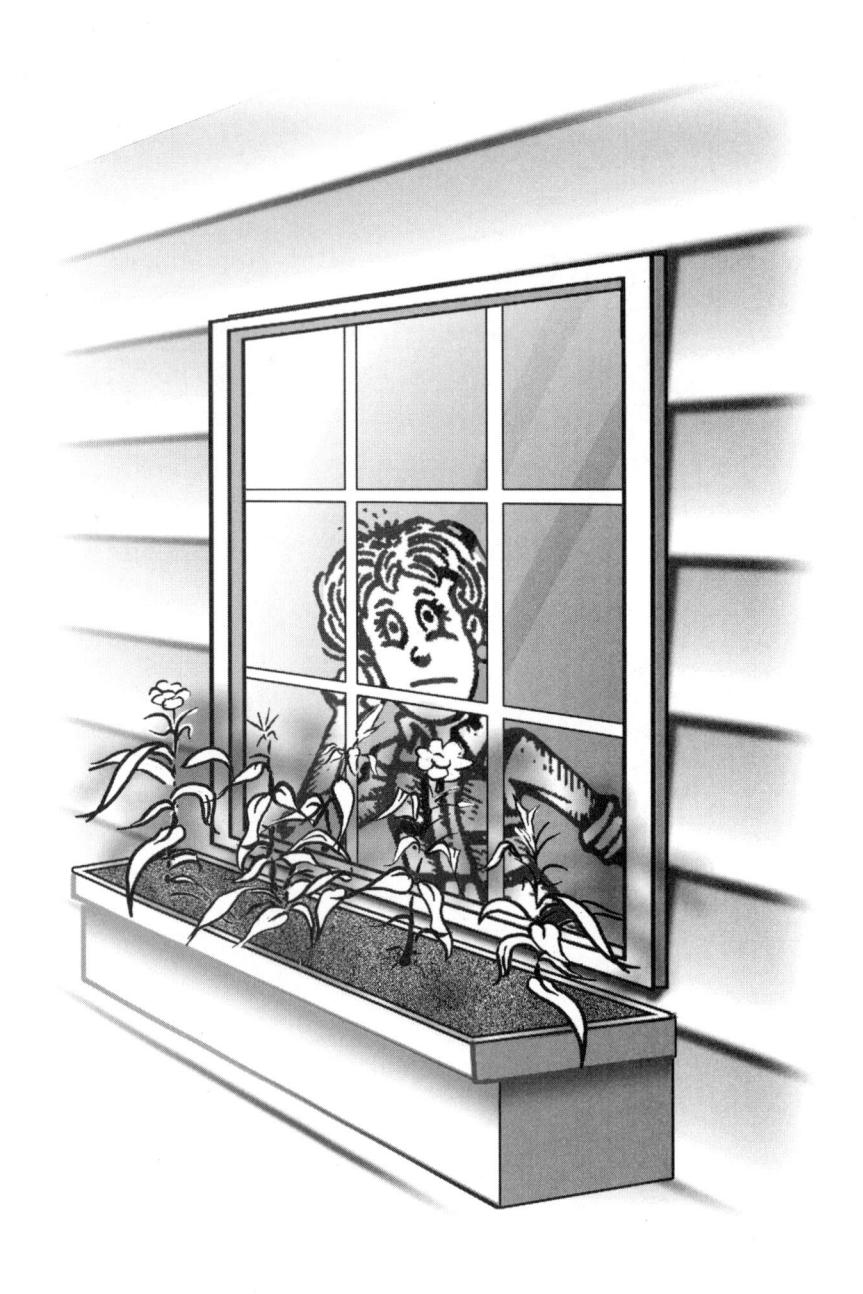

BLUE IS JUST ANOTHER COLOR

>Blues came walking in my room, I said,
>"Blues, please tell me what you are doing
>to make me feel so blue"?
>They looked at me and smiled, but refused to say.
>I seen them again and they turned and walked away.
>
>*"Rambling Blues"*
>*Ida Cox*

Whatever the reason for the arrival of the blues, Ida knew they would eventually turn and walk away. And since you're reading this book, you have been around long enough to understand the wisdom in her words. The blues wax and wane to our own internal tides. Women have EXPERIENCE with these visitors.

Do not impose your melancholia on the entire world. And it's not necessary to be a victim of emotional vagrancy by suffering in white knuckle silence. An old and precious friend is the best company when transacting with the blues.

We highly recommend calling your best pal. Admit we are in a bad mood to someone who won't hold it against you at a later date. Identify where it's coming from and deal with it. Express yourself, cry and curse. Be a big baby. She will understand. You'll get the chance to hold her hand some day.

Let's keep this among ourselves where the empathy levels are high. Share with sisters in transition. We know when the blues finally lift, we are welcomed back by other WITS to the sunny side of the street without recrimination. As with all support groups, it's best to share with those who "have been there."

"Friendship is all things shared."
Sue Gilmartin

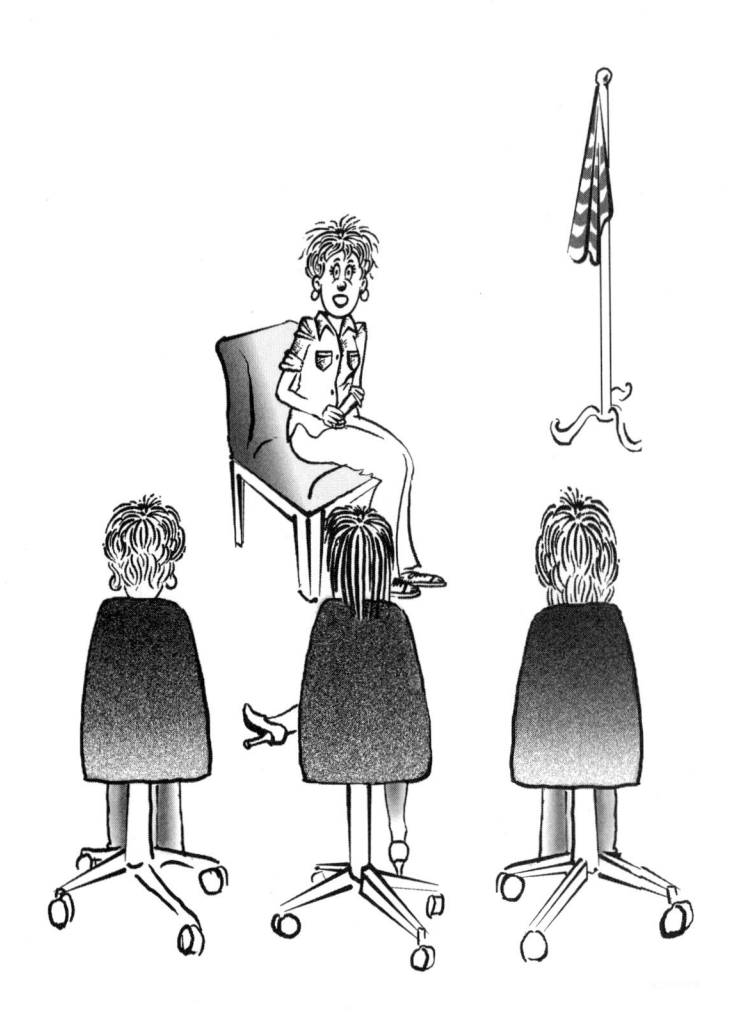

8

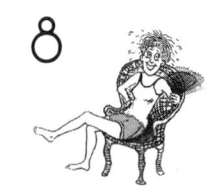

YOU ARE WHAT YOU THINK

Self-talk is like the evening news. It is chronically negative. And like the news, it is filled with information on disasters, past, present and future, and accompanied by the opinions of experts.

Our self-talk experts sit on a psychic Board of Directors who process all incoming data. Board members sort data into three major categories:

1. Grudges, past and present.

2. Injustices, revisited and yet to come.

3. Unworthiness, historical and current.

No data is ever discarded and new data is added every day. Over the years, this data base becomes the source of our self-talk. It takes on a life of its own. And it is lethal.

Looking for scientific verification of the Self-Talk Committee, we asked our friend, Sunny, to record her major thoughts for one day. Here is her daily diary:

6:00 a.m.   SHOWERING - Told off boss for lack of appreciation.

	Fantasized quitting job in a blaze of glory, leaving the boss and entire office staff dazzled.
7:15 a.m.	APPLYING MAKEUP - Entered a fugue state and relived breakup with former lover. Became teary-eyed. Ruined mascara.
7:45 a.m.	DRIVING TO WORK - Opinionated on other drivers. Hated other drivers. Vengefully tailgated, muttered threats. "That's it, Bub, make my day."
8:30-12 noon	LEARNING NEW SOFTWARE PROGRAM - Persistent messages of discouragement from the Committee. Cacophony of internal voices shrieking: "GIVE UP." "BLAME THE BOSS." "SMASH THE COMPUTER."
12:30-1:30 p.m.	ATE FIVE TACOS. More messages: "FOOD IS LOVE." "FORGET ABOUT HEART DISEASE." "SCREW OBESITY." "HAVE DESSERT."
1-5 p.m.	SUNK INTO A DEPRESSION. Had indigestion. Waistband painfully cutting into stomach. Messages of self-recriminations. Attempts to blame fellow workers for anything and everything.
5:30 p.m.	DRIVING HOME. See 7:45 a.m.
7-11 p.m.	COMATOSE IN FRONT OF TV. Ate potato chips and ice cream. Watched images of shapely 20 year olds working out, driving hot cars, falling in love, getting rich. Constant inner chant, "I HATE MYSELF."

    11-12 midnight TOSSED AND TURNED IN BED. Alternately hot and cold. Cursed menopause, facial wrinkles and the entire US Senate.

Sunny must ask herself, "Who exactly is in charge here?" Unfortunately, in Sunny's brain, the Committee reigns supreme.

Now, the Self-Talk Committee is not a phenomenon peculiar to middle-aged women. What is peculiar is that after 40+ years, we still allow this board of creeps to live rent-free in our minds.

The truth is we can only hold one thought in our minds at a time. We cannot rant and rave in the shower at our supposed enemies if we are singing "Me and Bobby McGee". We will not be just another crazed nut on the highway if we visualize the other driver as our best friend.

And what about learning new skills? If our value is "Intellect over Emotion", we can enjoy the learning process, be patient and applaud our accomplishments. In our middle years, we are more—not less—capable of learning new concepts.

As for over-eating and the TV? Hey, who needs it?

Finally, age and menopause are not the originators of our pain. Blame the Committee. Like Sunny, just listen to their crap for 24 hours. We are sure you will want to fire them immediately. No golden retirement umbrellas. No returning as consultants. Just show them the door. Then—silence and the opportunity to recreate our inner lives to reflect our true selves. What a concept!

"There is nothing either good or bad, but thinking makes it so."
Shakespeare

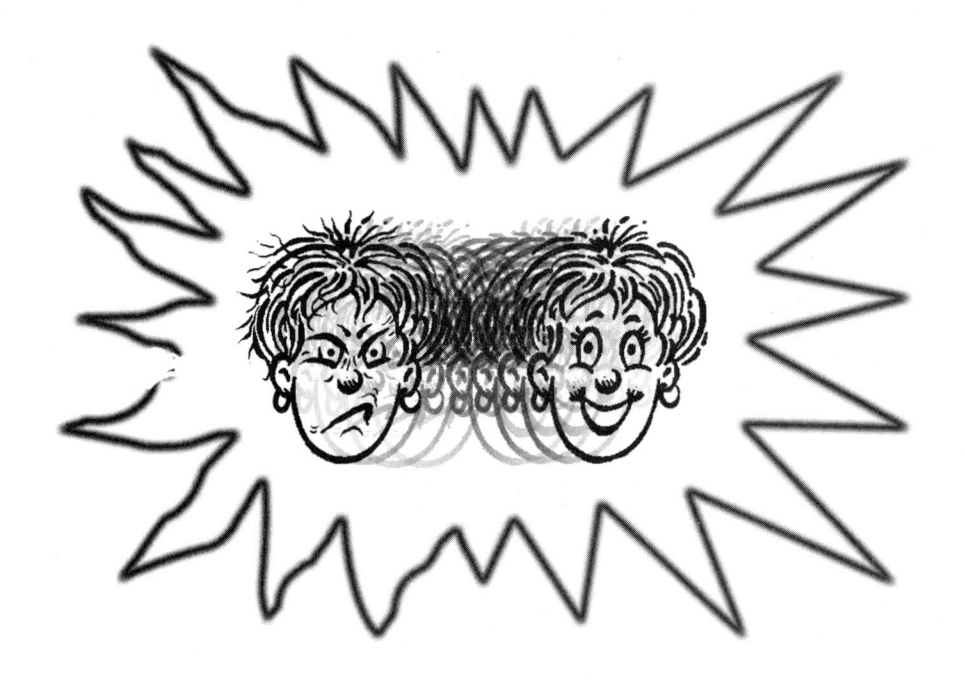

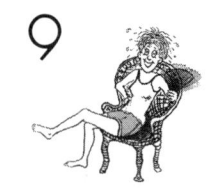

SLOWLY I TURN

Jeanette was in her husband's face—up close and personal. She hissed through gritted teeth, "Tell those damned painters to turn down that boom box or I'll turn it down for them!" Not waiting for a reply, she stormed out of the house. "Kill or be killed," she fumed. Her face was flushed, heart racing, palms sweaty. She was definitely on her last nerve.

Been there?? Done that??

We've examined this question of flashes of fury which seem to be quite common to women in their middle years. Unlike a therapist who might attribute this rage to childhood trauma, we are not interested in ancient history. We see the source of this rage as current. Not current as in time, but current as in electricity. Sister, this is a power surge. And the usually mild-mannered Jeanette is experiencing a mid-life blast of adrenaline straight from the hormones to her brain.

Power surges are not to be denied. However, if we direct them at others, homicide is a good possibility. And women's prison is no cakewalk. So these surges must be predicted and then deflected (to keep the world safe for others). It's important to recognize when we feel loaded and looking for a target. For example, a storm is brewing if our self-talk consists of the mantra, "I'm mad as hell and not going to take it anymore!" If we're about to smash—and we really mean smash—the Checker at WalMart, we must abandon our shopping cart and use the coming surge to propel us out the door. Best to clench our teeth and keep moving.

This is the truth of rage. It never works. Everything is in an exaggerated state. Words spoken in anger never persuade. Smashed dishes never mend. We see that it is in our own self-interest to ride the storm out in private. Take a breath, take a time out. Go for a walk. Find a private place and punch a pillow. Usually the emotion released after rage is sadness. So we often have a good cry. This might even be the time to have that peanut butter cookie you passed on last night. Then if we still have issues, we can address them in a calm and reasonable manner. Being calm and reasonable feels very good.

And Jeanette? She took one deep breath and marched past the painters and headed down the road. When she returned from a two-mile power walk, the painters were gone and her dignity was intact. However, she does plan to have a word with them next time.

"The unexamined life is not worth living."
Socrates

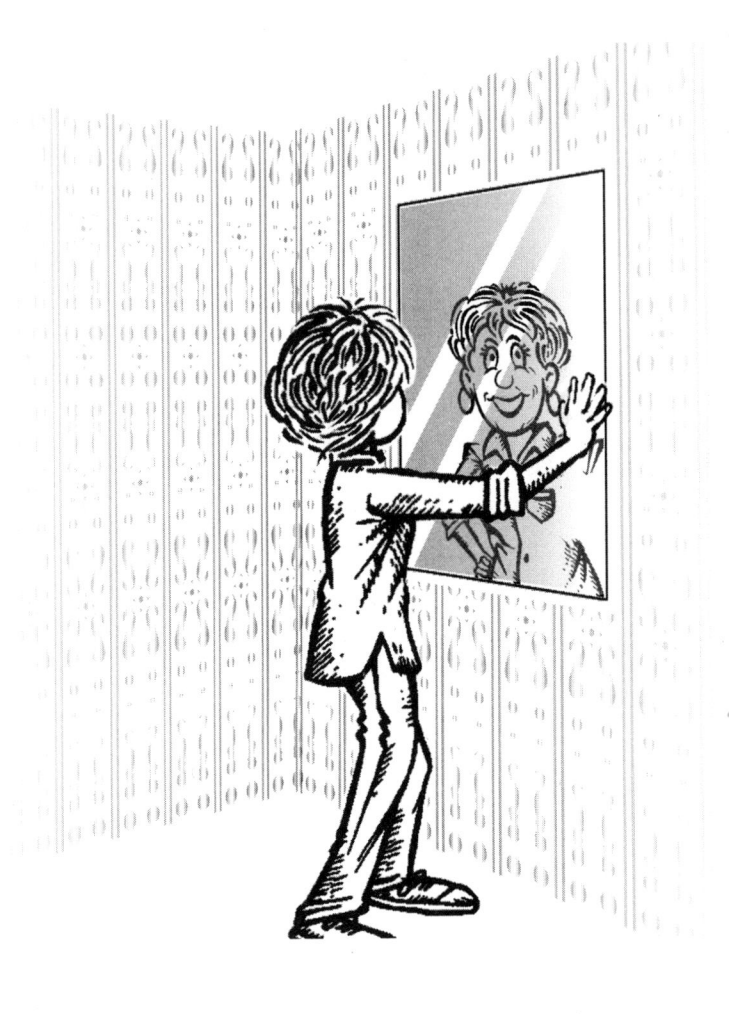

10

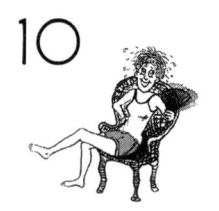

WHO, ME?

We get a kick out of the "real life" examples that appear in books and articles describing menopausal women. Here is a composite example of the fantasy which is held up to us as a reality!

> Marian, thin and fit at 52, is a successful clothes designer. Married to a famous Hollywood producer, 17 years her junior, Marian often socializes with the stars. Recently photographed with Brad Pitt, Marian fretted, "I look old enough to be his sister."

Hello! Who is this person?

She probably has shoes older than Brad. Well, maybe this woman exists in Hollywood, however, for the rest of us, facial wrinkles, graying hair and expanding waists are the norm.

The menopausal woman, as presented by the media, is a joke. Sadly, we all read about Marian, and assume we are the only ones who have not remained forever young.

What's wrong with aging with dignity and grace? Who cares if store clerks ask if we are buying the candy for our grandchildren? What's the matter with going to the weddings of our friends' children? Why not develop a model of beauty based on maturity, e.g., Lauren Bacall, Janet Reno, Elizabeth Dole, Ruth Gordon, Madeleine Albright, your best friend....

Whereas 100 years ago, most women were dead at 50, we are just beginning the second half of our lives. Interestingly, in some African societies, people do not know their ages because it is considered culturally insignificant. Well, it's time to come out of the closet—facial wrinkles and all. We are a "secret society" swelling in numbers. We have the power POLITICALLY AND FINANCIALLY. We can actually elect a President or put a sexist retailer out of business. We can start a country the size of Spain and Portugal combined.

Our sweatshirts read "50+ AND PROUD OF IT." Hey Marian, feeling a little left out?

"Resolve to be thyself; and know that he who finds himself loses his misery."
Matthew Arnold

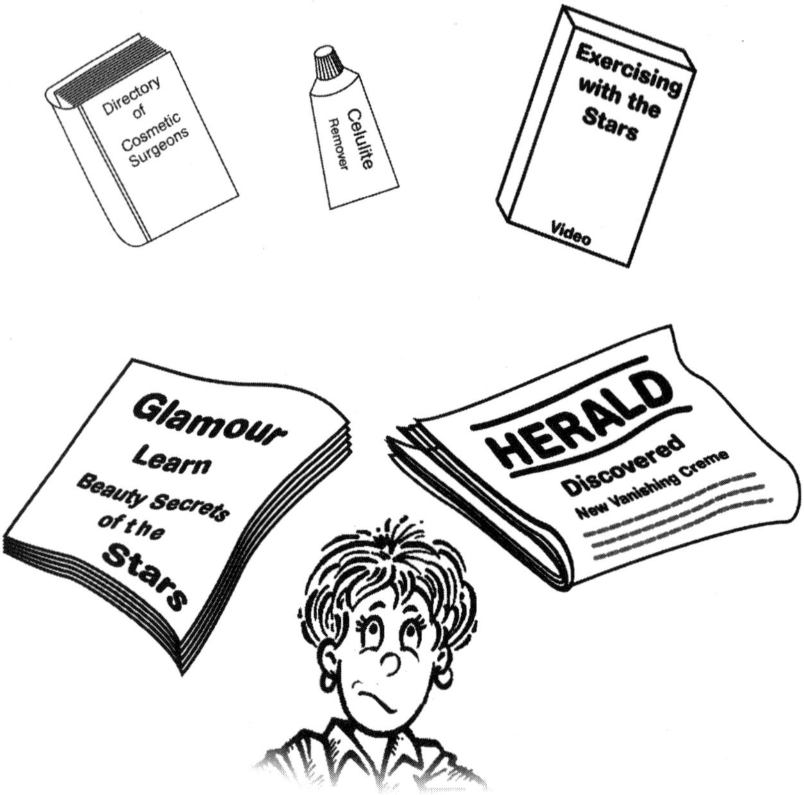
Directory of Cosmetic Surgeons
Celulite Remover
Exercising with the Stars
Video
Glamour
Learn Beauty Secrets of the Stars
HERALD
Discovered
New Vanishing Creme

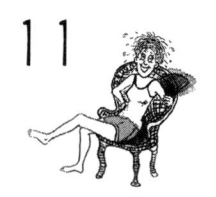

READ IT AND BLEEP @#$%*

The media is responsible for reporting the news. The news, and all other shows, are interspersed with brainwashing advertising. The political climate in Eastern Europe is given the same amount of time as an ad for Body Beautiful Gym. We get confused. We start to mix fact with fiction.

It's not easy to escape the media, (radio, TV, magazines, newspapers, junk mail, etc.) and its general adoration of youth and beauty. You know, the ads that urge you to hide the gray and camouflage wrinkles. Unfortunately, media shapes social attitudes.

Advertisers lead us to believe that without their products we will become menopausal pariahs. Their job is to instill in us the fear that on a specific day we will wake up in shapeless house dresses, body parts sagging. Our faces will crease up and grow warts. Our eyelids will flap, breasts droop, brains atrophy and buttocks fall behind our knees. On that fateful day, the Wrinkle Police will arrive at the front door, measure collagen levels and haul us off to Retirement City.

Sure, we don't look like we did when we were 21. In fact, we never had breasts that looked like a 1959 Oldsmobile bumper. When we were 21, plastic surgery was something that one had only after a near-fatal accident.

Anyway, good news on the doorstep is that we don't think like we did at 21 (thank God for big favors).

The media message is "Young is Best", but best for whom? At 50, we don't want to play volley ball in a thong bikini with a group of beer-drinking 20-year olds. They might be having an age-appropriate great time. However, we remember where all that sun-soaked frivolity led us—ridiculous behavior, projectile vomiting, three-day hangover and repair of reputation. This experience may be appropriate for passage into adulthood. However, the image of a middle-aged woman passed out on someone's front lawn doesn't seem real appealing. Know when you've stayed too long at the fair, regardless of media hype.

The reality is that this passage will occur with or without our permission. If you think you can bypass it, my friend, you are punching your ticket to Disappointment City. Sure, there are products on the market that do help us maintain an attractive self image. But don't forget, self-esteem is mainly an inside job.

"Age is something that doesn't matter unless you're a cheese."
Billie Burke

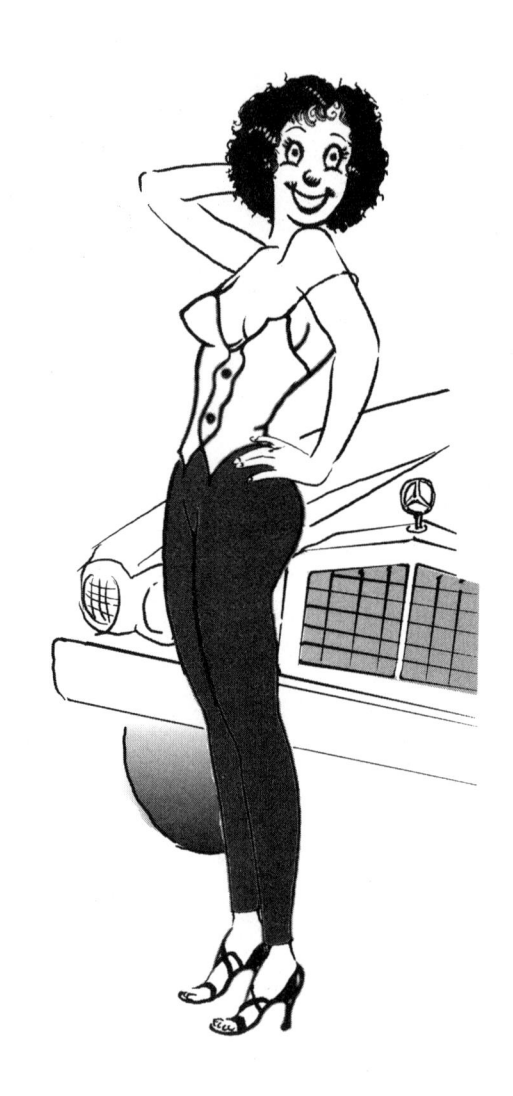

12

✗GET REAL!

Our friend, Rose, is a masseuse at a spa in Santa Monica, CA. She is often surprised, NO—shocked, when a 45 year-old woman comes through the door, and a 60 year-old body shows up at the massage table. Face and body just aren't a matching set. (Age assessments and actual age vary).

The point is that some women are hanging onto the idea of youthful looks with major fervor. Unless "Bodylift In a Jar" is discovered, lyposuction and plastic surgery will have to be part of their yearly OB/GYN regimen.

Without naming specific celebrities, we have observed that some aging actresses' eyes are continually moving closer to their ears. This phenomena is generally caused by the skin being pulled so tight so many times, that eventually the eyes appear to get farther and farther away from the front of the face. They look like frightened wall-eyed flounders. We do not exaggerate.

Rose also prides herself on being able to spot a facelift/eyelift from across the symphony hall. She can tell you how many surgeries have been performed. Some, she informs us, have had so many surgeries they can no longer close their eyes or move their mouths. This isn't bad if you're looking into another career as a ventriloquist. When we last talked with Rose about this subject, she said she's now in the process of being able to identify surgery by doctor.

We have seen women with so many nips and tucks that they look as if they are flying on the wing of the Concorde, and breast implants that undoubtedly could win an Oscar for "best special effects." Aren't they afraid they could hurt their grandchildren with those things?

The challenge of keeping the face and body matching can be a grueling life's work. We have observed some women who have expended their money and energy on body lifts to the exclusion of the face.

These women often dress in stiletto heels, halter tops and tight pants. From the back, they look very youthful with full manes of blonde hair (reminiscent of Farrah Fawcett in her nipple days). Once viewed from the front, however, it's REAL apparent REAL fast that this chick is well over 50. This look is okay if she's planning to walk backwards into rooms for the rest of her life.

Helene Deutsch, Freud's mentor, suggested that menopause triggers a return to the behavior patterns of adolescence. Although the contemporary glamorization of youth might provoke this behavior, she attributed it to "narcissistic self-delusion". You go, Helene.

"There's nothing wrong with being 50, unless you try to look 25."
(Joe Gillis to Norma Desmond in SUNSET BOULEVARD)

Confession#1: Love that Vitamin E Cream!

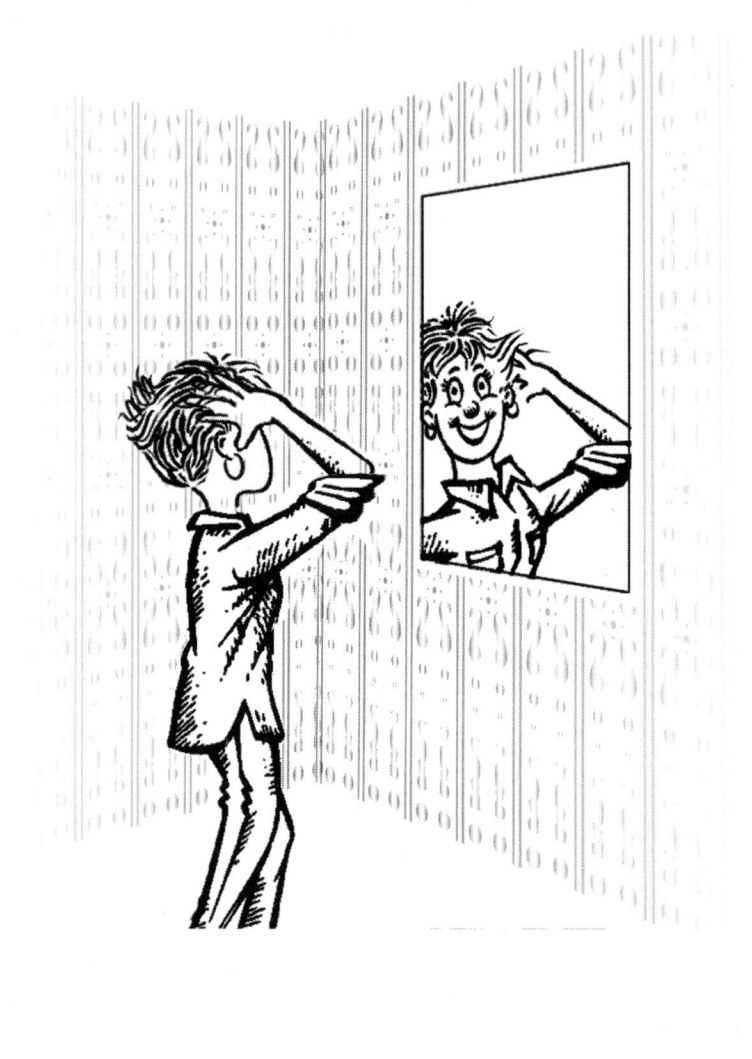

MIRROR, MIRROR ON THE WALL

Pat squirts hair spray on all three mirrors in her bathroom. And we know why. The better <u>not</u> to see you, my dear. This is her way of negotiating with vanity.

Hey, Pat, try this: Look into a clean mirror (yeah, include the chin and neck) and make eye contact. Okay, shoulders back. Breathe deeply. Smile with confidence. Feel good. Now chant one of the following until you are happy with who you see:

Lookin' good, girl.

It could be worse.

Hi, Mom.

Whatever works. The point is this: You look okay. Hey, you probably look beautiful. It's all in the eye of the beholder and you are the one beholding.

> *"There is no cosmetic for beauty like happiness."*
> *Anonymous*

Confession#2: We don't own any magnifying mirrors.

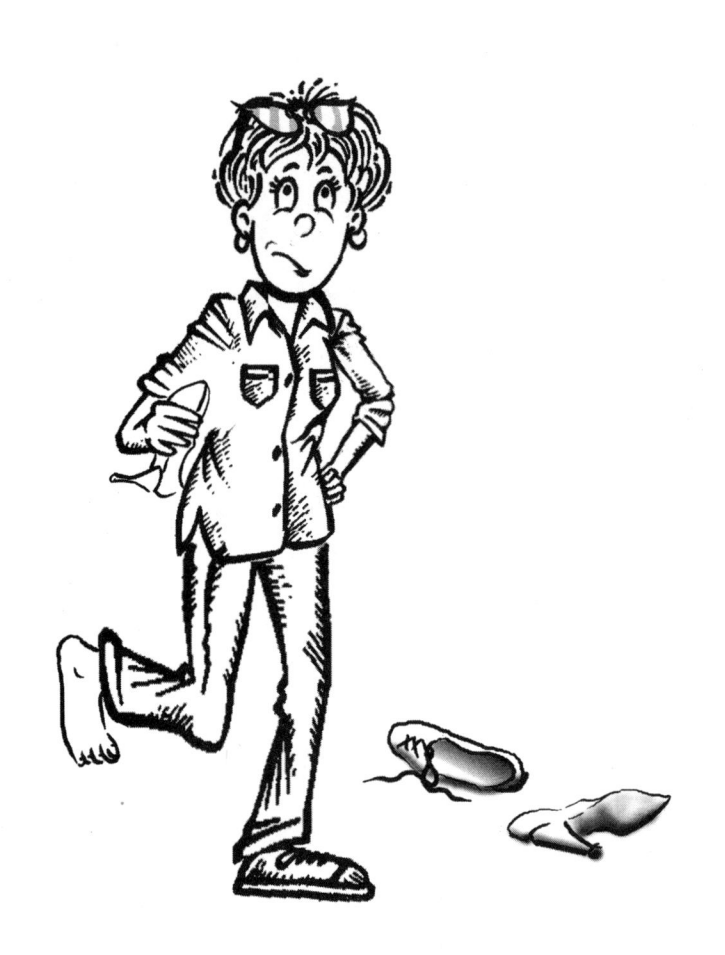

14

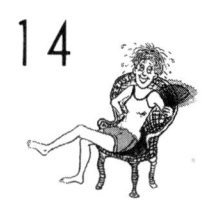

MORE ON MEMORY LOSS

We are continually losing nouns, events, and occasions. Simple words escape us, but who cares? We are masters at making up words and sentences.

When asking a friend if she's busy, it's not unusual for her to blurt out, "Up to my earballs." And we know what she means, right? Then there are times when speaking to a coworker, we have had to glance at her name plate to remember her name.

Simple words escape us. You left your wallet in...the supermarket?... San Francisco?... The word could very well be CAR. Those three-letter words will get you every time.

We congratulate ourselves for being organized until we find a sponge in the refrigerator. Who knows when it was left there and only God knows what should have been in its place. Is a head of broccoli under the sink?

And we are especially fond of all the notes we make to ourselves to be sure not to forget anything. You know, the post-it which reads "Remember appointment with what's-her-name." When we get around to reading it, we have no idea what it means. Then a day later we find that we've missed a doctor's appointment. Ah, so that's what the note meant.

We have a very pithy comment about a movie recently seen. Unfortunately, when we can't remember the name, who starred in it, or what it's about, the comment "well worth seeing" carries little weight.

We have observed that a new talent generally comes to the forefront at this time of our lives. We have the ability to tell entire stories with hand, eye and brow movements, with little or no talking. Perhaps a grunt here or there. And what's more, most of our friends know exactly what we mean.

This isn't as bad as it sounds because there is sure to be a lot of stuff we're all happy to forget. If, in the sea of lost memories, the title of a movie floats away, so be it.

We did have some solutions—but we forgot them. You might not remember them anyway.

"There is only one great adventure; inwards, towards the self."
Henry Miller

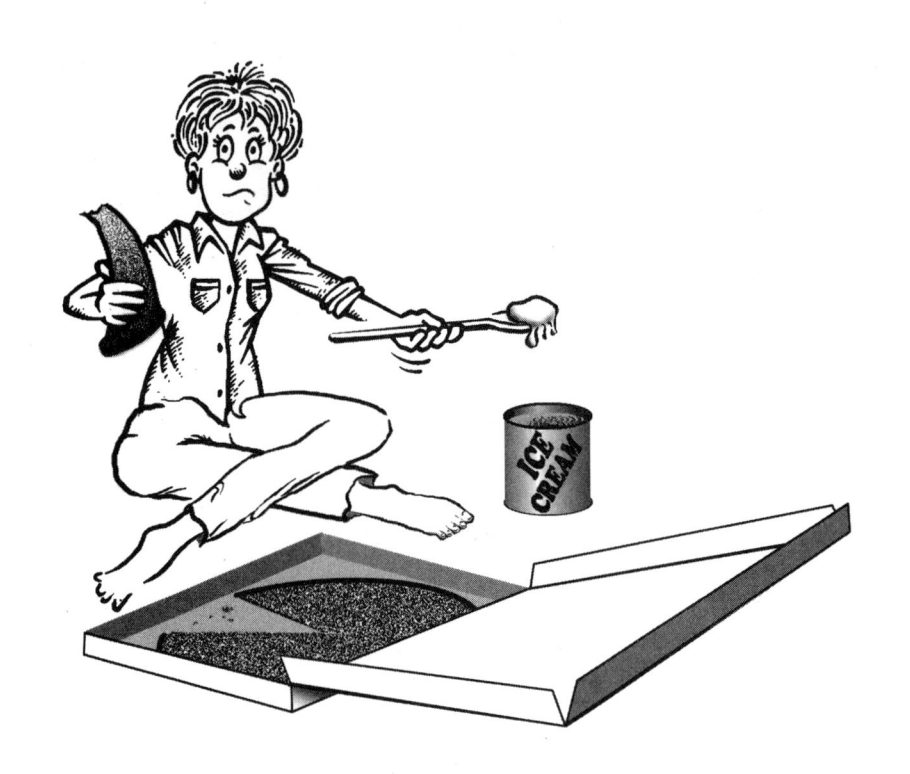

15

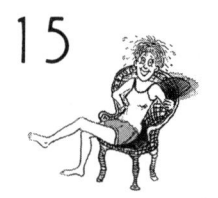

LARGER THAN LIFE

The word has been passed down through the generations that once you hit 40, it's much harder to lose weight. True. Weight maintenance may be more difficult because we tend to exercise less, metabolism changes and so on. However, unless we are satisfied to get our clothes from Omar the Tentmaker, we have to be more mindful of what and when we eat.

Now there are three ways to go with weight gain:

>Give up.

>Throw up.

>Grow up.

We opt for the third alternative which, incidentally, will provide for some good role modeling for our daughters, granddaughters and those we choose to mentor. By "grow up" we mean a simple application of the Serenity prayer.

<u>Accept the Things We Cannot Change:</u> Do you find yourself saying things like, "I'm a size 5 if it's cut big"? WHAT DOES THAT MEAN??

It probably means you're not a 5 (duh). Stop shopping in juniors, buy comfortable clothes, especially skirts with a realistic waist size.

<u>The Courage to Change the Things We Can:</u> We really don't need two giant-sized peanut butter cookies at 3 in the morning. This we can change. Be brave—write down everything you eat for a week. You will soon know why, even 3 hours after you've taken off your jeans, it still looks like you're wearing them. We can tell each other, "I hardly eat anything," but a weekly food list will always reveal the truth.

This is not a lecture on diets. After all, we are the generation who buys all the diet books and participates in all the diet programs. We've made diet book authors wealthy and famous. We've eaten cabbage soup, grapefruits or rice for weeks. Many of us own every jazzercize tape in the history of civilization. Granted, they've never been opened, but we own them nonetheless. Sound familiar?

<u>The Wisdom to Know the Difference:</u> If you have never been a size 5, why look to be one at age 47? Wisdom dictates be healthy, not delusional. Linda did tell us that when she got out of a steamy shower one morning and saw herself in the mirror, her first thought was, "Hey, who's in here with me?" It was then she decided to be more watchful of her eating habits.

When the child-within screams "CHOCOLATE," the adult-without wisely counsels "FRUIT." We feed both our child and adult without spoiling either.

"Life itself is the proper binge."

Julia Child

Confession Number 3: **We ate more than a dozen biscotti while writing this chapter.**

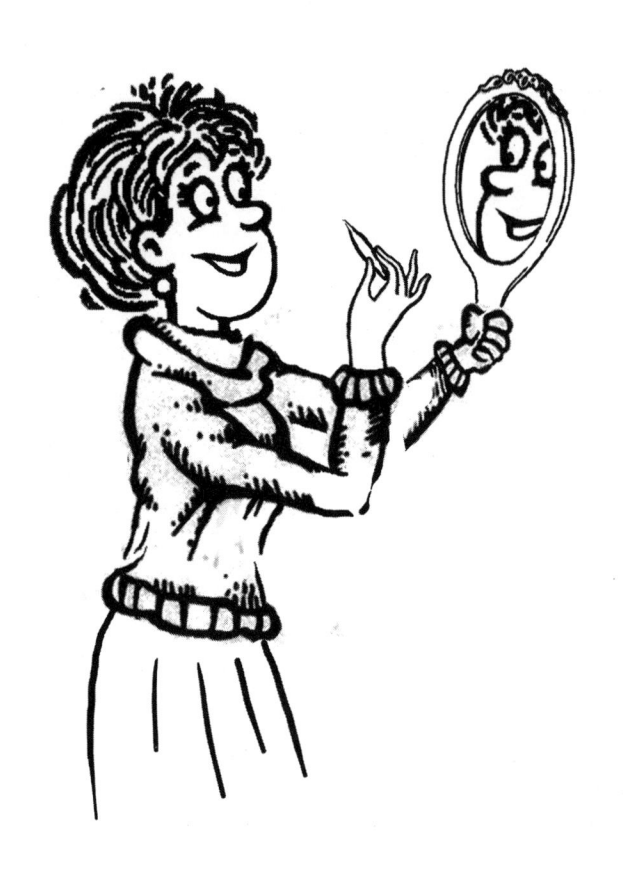

HAIR TODAY, HAIR TOMORROW

A strange phenomenon occurs during this period of life. As the hair on our legs seems to be more sparse, it starts to appear on our chins. You know, those little stubbles that you can't wait to tweeze. You are sure these follicles are hanging down at least to your waist. What's reassuring about this is that we can spot a "tweezer chin twin" from quite a distance away. (Unless, of course, you are having Visual Deficits, which are discussed later in this book.)

Nikki told of watching a talk show on national TV. A famous actress was discussing her new movie while caressing and assessing her chin hairs. There it was, right on TV, the secret handshake, the Honeymooners' Ralph Kramden/Ed Norton Raccoon Lodge signal, the club code. To women of mid-age this is the high sign of all high signs. Regardless of all other differences, Nikki could relate to those little black chin hairs.

Although we always think the world can spot the little buggers from across a football field, it's probably best, in public, to just make a mental note of their location. Once at home, follow this simple technique: locate and tweeze, locate and tweeze, using alternate hands in a rhythmic motion. This routine holds the seed of a Zen moment and may change your consciousness. Honest to God, your eyes will glaze over.

When you see a "tweezer chin twin," give her a smile and a nod. You've both been there and will continue to be there. Tweezing chin hairs is like housework, it's never done.

We have been searching for other than the above mentioned solution, and until now have come up with:

Waxing (ouch!)

Electrolysis (really ouch!)

Join circus (could be fun!—don't laugh)

It's noteworthy here to mention that Mother Nature is very fair and just. While the above situation occurs in women's lives, let us not forget that when men's hair starts to thin, it begins to appear more and more in their noses and ears.

One last important thing to remember, this is a good time to assign a friend to the duty of tweezing your chin hairs in the event you go into a coma. Here is an example of how this can be included in your Living Will:

I (_____) do solemnly swear that I will remove all chin hairs from (_____) in the event she becomes incapacitated/comatose and unable to tweeze on her own. I further promise that I will do this on an every other day basis for as long as we both shall live.

Signature

(Depending on level of trust, you may want to have this notarized.)

"I know by the hair on my chinny chin chin."
(from THE THREE LITTLE PIGS)

Choice

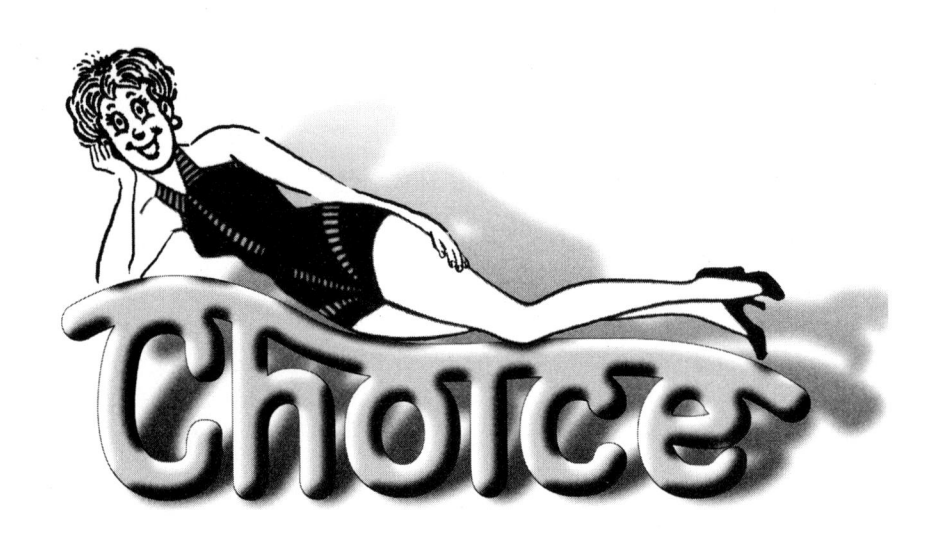

17

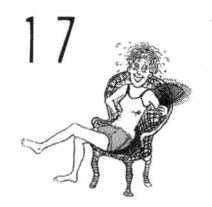

TO EACH HER OWN

Sex. We don't know what to tell you here. Some of our friends have become real nymphs, now that the kids are out of the house and there's no more fear of pregnancy. Others have been so active for so long, they're on sexual sabbatical or maybe full retirement.

There are no rules when it comes to sex except that it must be done with a consenting adult or inanimate object—your choice. Whatever you want is all right, cause you're all right.

"Sex is a Jungle."
Woman on "Northern Exposure"

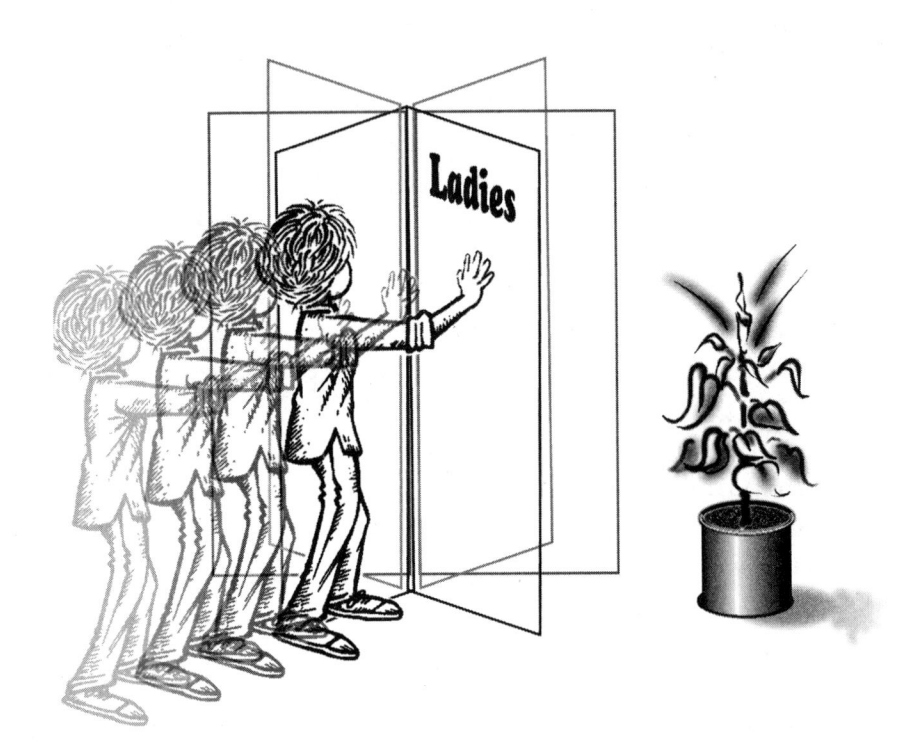

18

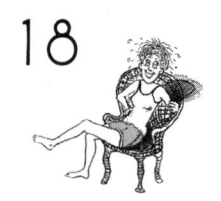

A RIVER RUNS THROUGH IT

Be careful jogging, sneezing, coughing, laughing, even breathing! Your bladder ain't what it used to be.

These days, no matter how many times we use the restroom before we leave our offices, we find that as soon as we pull onto our streets, and see the front door, our bladders are in charge. We often wonder if someone flashed a photograph of the front door if it would have the same effect. Similarly, on long car trips, why is it that everything is fine until we see the sign that reads "NEXT REST STOP—25 miles." We automatically panic because we know our bladders are only good for 18 miles.

These symptoms are reminiscent of childhood. Who doesn't remember the Potty Dance—running into the house, jumping up and down, stamping feet, and charging to the bathroom? All to the sound of Mom yelling, "Why do you always wait until the last minute?" At this point in life, how many of us heed Mom's words, "Be sure you go to the bathroom before you leave!" (C'mon, raise your hands, we know you're out there.)

Darnell tells us that she knows every bathroom facility in her sales territory. This information is essential to any WIT who leaves home. She has standards as to what is an acceptable rest stop and has rated them from one to five (five the best). She does admit that sometimes her bodily need wins over her snob appeal, and she will stop at a one.

Accidents do happen. A good friend, Ariel, was at a restaurant. Apparently, something became lodged in her throat, and she started to choke. As she told it, the outcome had GOOD news and BAD news. A knight in white armor had remembered his CPR training, specifically the Heimlich maneuver. He ran over to her table, lifted her from her chair, thrust his hands around her sternum and pounded away with all his might. The food was dislodged. This was the GOOD NEWS. The BAD NEWS? During the commotion, she wet all over her hero.

Insight might be gained here. First, listen to your mother. Be sure to use the bathroom before you leave... anywhere. Secondly, follow Darnell's lead. Even the funkiest rest stop is better than a wet car seat. Lastly, Ariel's experience may not win $100,000 on America's Funniest Home Videos, but we sure got a good laugh out of it. Hey, that's what it's about.

"Laugh and the World Laughs With You."
We're not sure who said this, maybe Queen Elizabeth

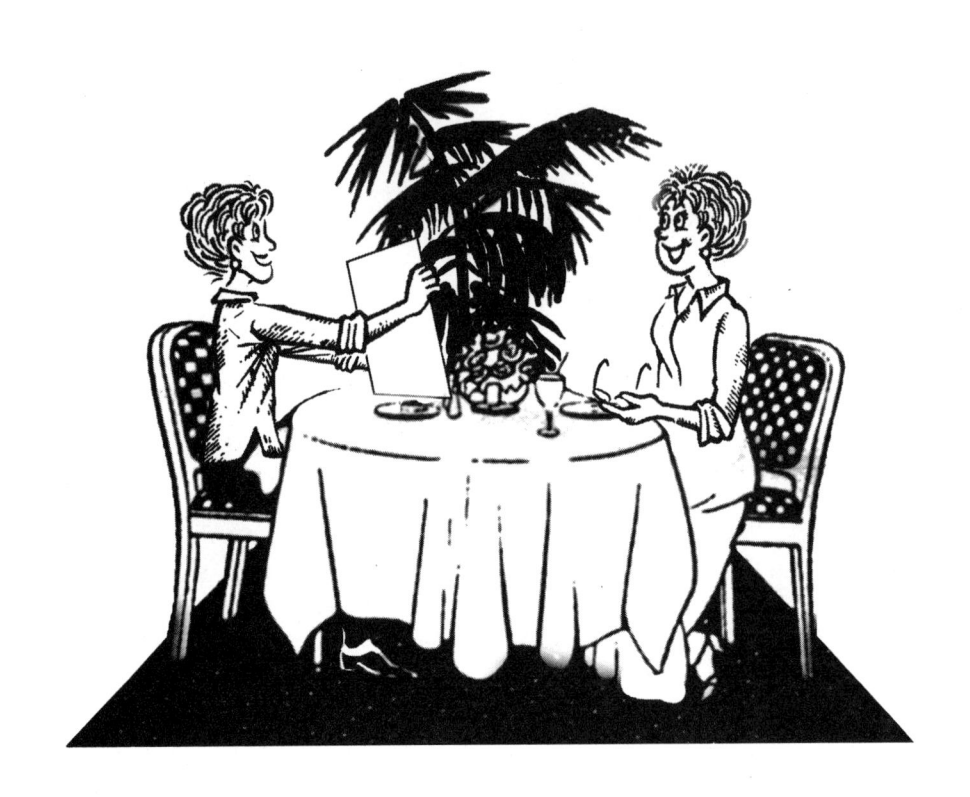

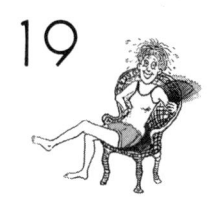

DO YOU SEE WHAT I SEE?

Since one of us is nearsighted and the other farsighted, we find it is prudent to travel together. The farsighted driver has her eye on the bigger picture. This includes the highway signs and identifying road kill. The nearsighted passenger keeps her eye on the map and speedometer, which gives her license to yell, "Slow down" or "Are you trying to get us killed?"

When we stop at restaurants, no problem. One holds the menu and the other reads it from across the table. Aren't we the solution-oriented ones?

The buddy system works especially well while playing Bingo. The nearsighted buddy can mark the Bingo cards, while the farsighted buddy reads the numbers from the board. This system works equally well at foreign movies. One reads the subtitles and the other sorts the Jujyfruits by color. Easy, no?

Once left to our own devices, we have individually found solutions to other typical optical problems. Have you noticed the print on product labels at the supermarket is getting smaller? Simply carry a magnifying glass. If you've been afflicted with memory loss that day (ergo, no magnifying glass), simply stop any person under 30 and assault them with questions. For example, "Would you show me which Fettucini Alfredo has the lowest fat content?" or "Which toilet tissue has more than 200 sheets per roll?"

So, Although we may be losing the keen eyesight of youth, by sharing the load, we are gaining a new way of seeing the world (pun intended).

"It is only with the heart that one can see rightly; what is essential is invisible to the eye."
Antoine de Saint-Exupery

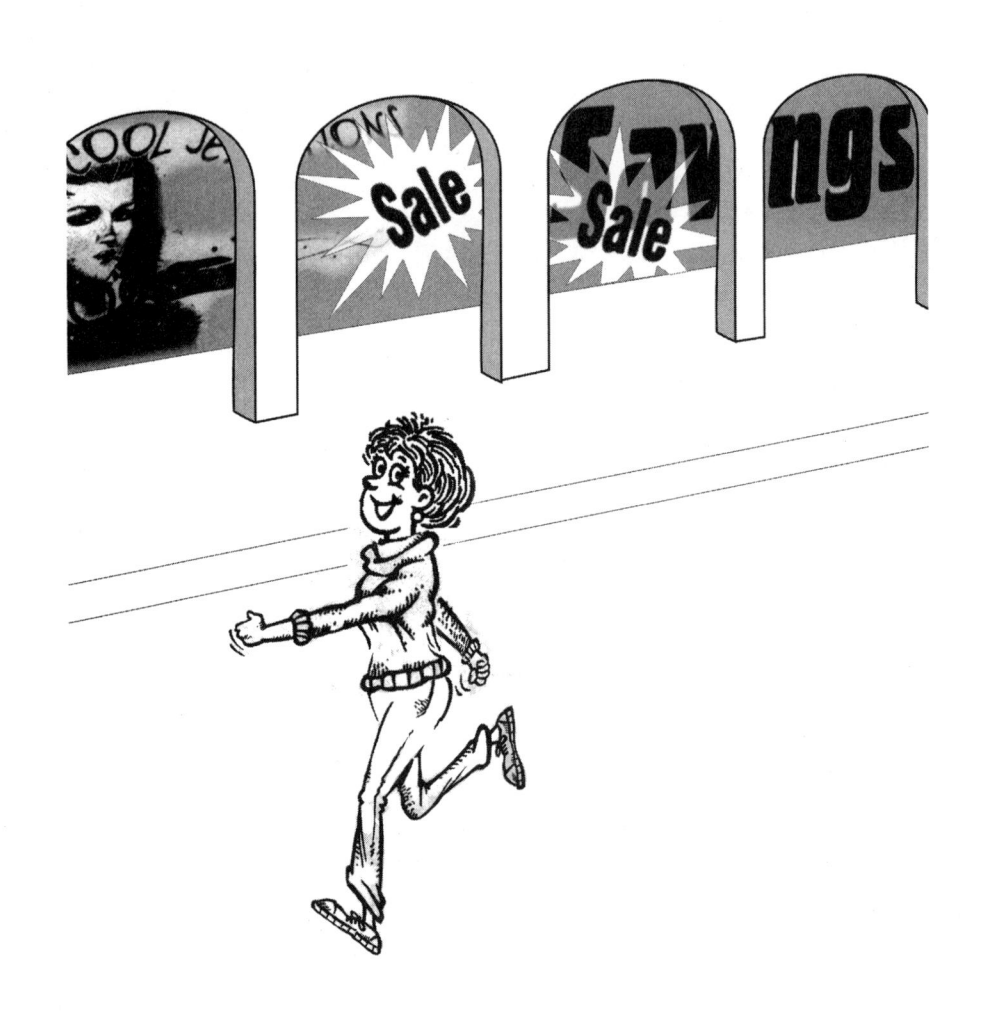

20

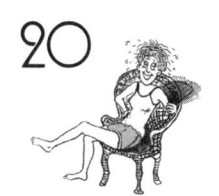

MALL MADNESS

Freud asked, "What do Women Really Want?" If he looked at our credit cards and closets, he might assume we want Stuff. Most of us suffer from "stuffitis" (materialism) big time. We use shopper's "high" and crammed closets to assure ourselves that we may be middle-aged, but we can buy whatever we damn well please.

Let's reevaluate the premise that stuff equals happiness. It may be a value imposed upon us by years of habit and media manipulation. Actually, as we take our position as wise and venerated elders, our need for material possessions will lessen. We will no longer be advising our sisters and daughters coming along the path to "Shop Like You Mean It" but rather to "Live Like You Mean It." Check out these comparisons between the MATERIAL GIRL and the MINIMALIST WOMAN and decide for yourself who you would rather be in these middle years.

MATERIAL GIRL	MINIMALIST WOMAN
Hoards goods.	Donates regularly and generously.
Cruises the mall armed with	Power walks the mall

new credit cards.	with no credit cards.
Gets high purchasing.	Gets high walking on the beach.
Goes to all sales.	Goes to all art openings.

Moving from a shopping savant to a spiritual path is as easy as practicing one of the principles of Minimalist Woman. Sure, we enjoy cruising the frou-frou shops and garage sales, but some things can't be purchased. For example, good conversation. When we go to the mall together, we do some shopping, lots of laughing, solve some problems and maybe come up with a few new ideas. This isn't a lecture on resistance, but our statement on balance.

"We work to become, not acquire."
E. Hubba

Confession Number 4: Shoes! Gotta have them!

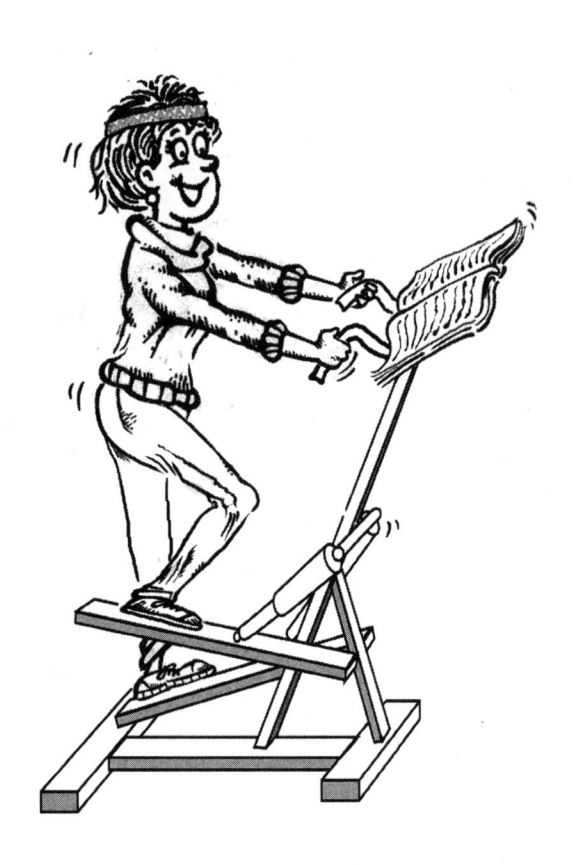

21

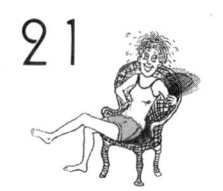

SCHOOL DAZE

Robin sat across from the College Admissions Director sunk in despair. "Five years of night school to get a degree," she moaned, "I'll be 52 years old before I finish!" The Admissions Director eyeballed Robin and replied, "Well, chances are you will be 52 in five years anyway. Do you want to be 52 with or without a degree?" DUH!

Going back to school in the middle years can be a scary proposition. We doubt our intellectual ability to learn, we dread failure, we question our physical stamina to endure the long haul. In other words, we hate to leave our comfort zone. However, for those of us brave enough to take on higher education, the rewards are enormous.

Robin decided to override her fear and enroll in school. By the time she completed the registration process, she thought she may have gotten a Physics Major with a Ballet Minor, but she persevered. The first class was confusing. She was overwhelmed by the course material. She could not remember how to take notes. She was tired. The occasional hot flash did not help. Yet, she endured by chanting "One Day at a Time" to and from the campus.

After several months, Robin was in the groove. Once she relaxed, she noticed several other WITS in the class. She made friends and formed a Study Group. A whole new dimension of life was opening up to her: Academia. Here facial wrinkles and expanding waists were of little interest to women who were debating economic theory or mastering Computer Graphics. Now her "dead-end" job became the vehicle which allowed her to pay for school. Robin now had a different future.

And you better believe it—there is a future. With good health habits, we will lead productive lives for another 25 or 30 years. So what are we going to do with all that time on our hands? We can just spend so much time shopping and applying face creams. Would you like to be known as someone who had cute outfits or someone who enjoyed and used her brain? Or both?

Exercising the brain is just as rewarding as exercising on a stair master. In fact, Robin now does both at the same time. She props up her textbook on Time Management and pumps away. The vital juices begin to flow both physically and intellectually. This is empowerment.

"You either change things or you don't."
Agnes Whistling Elk

83

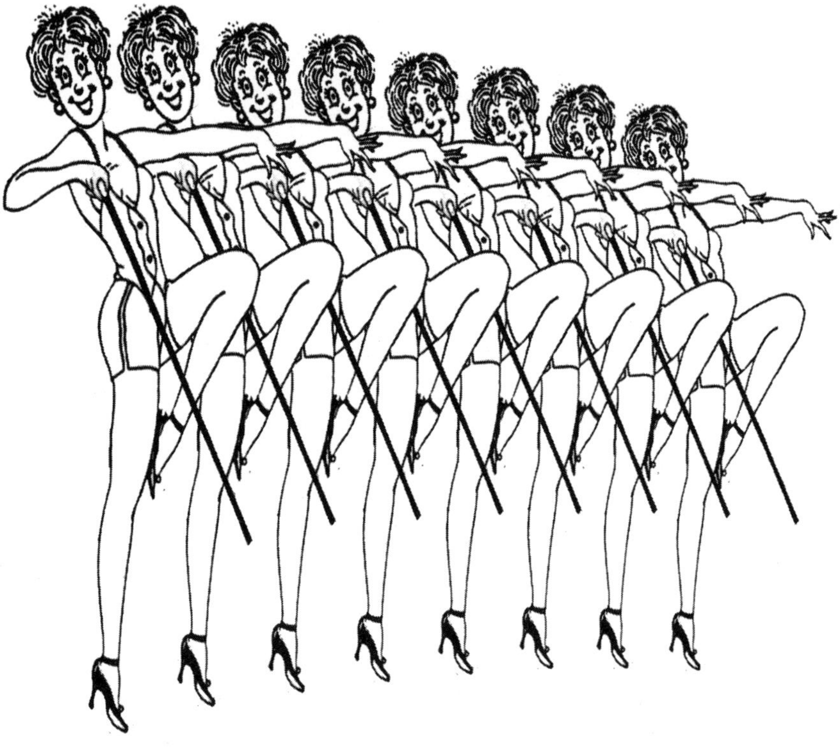

SOFT SHOE FOR THE SOUL

There are two groups of people renowned for talking aloud—the mentally challenged and menopausal women.

We saw Millie in the video store carrying on an animated conversation. As we approached her, we caught the tail end of her comments, "Oh yeah, that was a great film—too bad I saw it already—gotta get popcorn." We looked for her companion. (A large white rabbit maybe?) However, Millie was definitely alone.

Now we know Millie's mental health is okay. We also know she turned 51 last year. That makes Millie a menopausal mutterer. Is this bad? We think not. Does it matter that some people may think she's been beamed in from another planet? Another resounding, we think not. Actually, the ability to shock people is life-enhancing and funny. It's essential to good mental health to do something ridiculous daily.

By the time we've reached our middle years, most of us are discovering we enjoy conversing aloud with ourselves. In many cultures, individuals who talk to themselves, even spontaneously sing and dance, are considered Shamen or wise persons. They are not considered mentally ill, but rather bursting with inner vision. So, too, with menopausal women. Hey, we cannot keep all that energy contained for the purpose of social decorum.

And just like Shamen, singing and dancing become part of our celebration of life. Gail was recently reported dancing in the aisles of WalMart. Helene talks to herself so often that her family constantly interjects, "Just let us know when you want us to jump in here."

Are these forms of self-expression any less valid than body piercing? It may be our age bias, but we would rather see a woman doing an imitation of Ginger Rogers than a girl with gold studs in her tongue.

Wouldn't it be a lovely world if it were commonplace to see women breaking into song and dance in public settings? We envision a rainy morning, everyone intent on getting to the office. As the crowd surges across the street, one woman begins humming "Singing in the Rain." Another joins in, adding a few dance steps. These two are joined by four more. Each of them is twirling her umbrella and singing, "What a glorious feeling, I'm happy again!" Now the six of them two-step across the street, joined by six more, voices soaring, feet tapping. The rest of the crowd parts and watches in awe. Twelve middle-management, middle-aged women turning a dreary morning into a magical moment. Gene Kelly would be proud.

Well, why not? We are so great in numbers that acting in concert we can do whatever we damn well please. If our individual energy is added to that of other WITS, we could give concerts that even rock-stars would envy. We could also lobby to change laws, raise money for AIDS research, cure cancer, visit every lonely hospitalized child. We are at that great jumping off point into the second half of our lives where anything is possible. Let's make our voices heard either in song or in community debate. Just don't get arrested. It's not middle-age cool.

"Don't compromise yourself, you're all you've got."
Janis Joplin

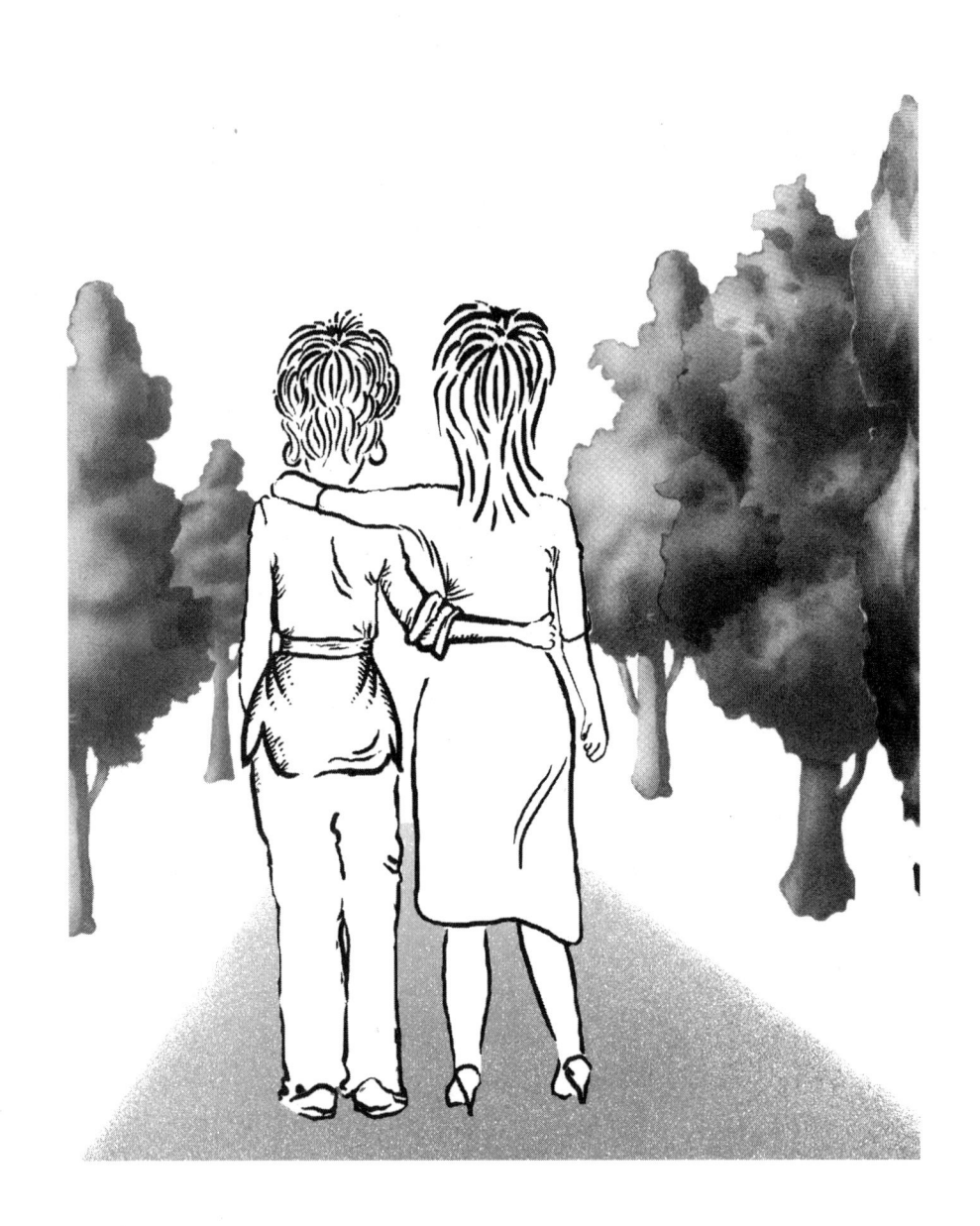

23

WRAP UP

Menopausal symptoms are the wake-up call.

During menopause, there is a natural expression of personal power and wisdom available to women. It's a time when one can find a deeper and freer experience of self. This high level of personal power can be used for purposes that serve not only ourselves but others as well.

We are in the position of revering this time as the renaissance of the middle years. After years of bumbling through, it's now time to take stock. The clouds have parted and we can clearly see the person that is emerging.

Auntie Mame quipped, "Life is a smorgasbord and most poor suckers are starving to death." Grace Slick advises, "Feed your head." Both of these WITS have the right idea.

The following delicacies are available at life's smorgasbord and are guaranteed to feed your head... and your heart:

> Send love letters to J. D. Salinger—what the heck, he won't answer them anyway.

Plant a vegetable garden.

Flaunt wearing white pants.

Run for office.

Bay at the moon.

Write a song.

Go river rafting.

Wear chartreuse shoes.

Place pictures of you and friends throughout the house.

Plant a garden.

Tear into gifts.

Tutor a child.

Send pictures of you as a child to everyone you know.

Hug often.

Learn another language.

Go on a game show.

Take tango lessons.

Have a funeral for the old you.

Schedule quiet time for yourself.

Cherish companions/friends.

Yell, "I Rule!".

**Feel deeply—enjoy simply—take risks—be yourself.
Good friends—Good support—Good diet—Good luck!**

"During menopause, the flow of energy becomes intensified and steady like a direct current. We are charged with energy to the degree we have opened ourselves to the wisdom of the crone."
Farida Sharan